The Hypothyroidism Diet

Delicious recipes

Author

Frances D. Hall

Green Beans and Sesame-Crusted Tuna Rosemary Cauliflower and Roasted Pork Mexican Soup in a Flash

- Soup with Fresh Basil and Roasted Tomatoes

- Soup made with turkey sausage, butternut squash, and kale Dessert Cups in Chocolate

- Chocolate Frosting with buttercream Homemade Chocolate Caramelized Hazelnut Spread

- Sprinkled Coconut Whipping Cream of Coconut

- Eggs, Veggies, and Parmesan on a Sheet Pan

- Cheddar-Stuffed Burgers With Zucchini Grilled Pesto Salmon With Asparagus With Cauliflower Sesame Chicken Cordon Bleu -Green Beans and Tuna Crusted Rosemary Cauliflower and Roasted Pork Mexican Soup in a Flash

- Delicious Italian Vegetable Soup with Roasted Tomatoes and Fresh Basil

- Soup made with turkey sausage, butternut squash, and kale Cauliflower Soup in Tuscan Style

- Cheesy Broccoli Soup In A Bread Bowl Shrimp & Cod Stew In Tomato-Saffron Broth Fudge with chocolate Ripple\sBacon Chunks of ripe sour cherry Curd with Lemons Drops of pb

- Cabbage Casserole with Low-Carb Zucchini and Walnut Salad with Low-Carb Broccoli Mash

- Macaroni and Cauliflower

- Bacon and balsamic vinegar Vegetable Soup with a Medley of Vegetables from the Garden

- Pecan Cookie with Blueberries Muffin Cake

- Asparagus Broccoli, Bacon, and Cheese Hash with Cauliflower granola quiche

Introduction

The thyroid is a small butterfly-shaped gland that sits just below the Adam's apple at the base of your neck. The endocrine system is a complex network of glands. Many of your body's activities are controlled by the endocrine system. Hormones that regulate your body's metabolism are made by the thyroid gland.

When your thyroid produces too much (hyperthyroidism) or not enough (hypothyroidism), it can cause a variety of problems (hypothyroidism).

Hyperthyroidism

Thyroid gland is overactive in hyperthyroidism. It makes an excessive amount of the hormone it produces. About one percent of women have hyperthyroidism. Men have a lower prevalence of it.

Graves' disease is the most common cause of hyperthyroidism, affecting approximately 70% of those who have an overactive thyroid. Thyroid nodules, also known as toxic nodular goiter or multinodular goiter, can cause the gland to produce too much hormone.

Symptoms of increased thyroid hormone production include: • restlessness

• jitters • irritability • racing heart

• a greater tendency to sweat

• shaking

Anxiety, insomnia, and thin skin are some of the symptoms of anxiety.

• hair that is brittle, as well as nails that are brittle.

• a lack of muscle

• Loss of body weight

• Graves' disease causes bulging eyes.

Diagnosis and therapy for hyperthyroidism

Thyroid hormone (thyroxine, or T4) and thyroid-stimulating hormone (TSH) levels in the blood can be determined with a blood test. TSH is a hormone released by the pituitary gland to stimulate thyroid hormone production. Your thyroid gland is overactive if your thyroxine levels are high and your TSH is low.

Your doctor may also administer radioactive iodine to you orally or intravenously, and then monitor how much your thyroid gland absorbs. Iodine is required for the production of hormones by your thyroid. Thyroid overactivity is indicated by a high level of radioactive iodine in your system. The low level of radioactivity dissipates quickly, and the majority of people are unaffected.

The thyroid gland is destroyed or prevented from producing hormones in hyperthyroidism treatment.

Antithyroid drugs like methimazole (Tapazole) stop the thyroid from making hormones.

The thyroid gland is harmed by a high dose of radioactive iodine. It is taken by mouth as a pill. When your thyroid gland absorbs iodine, it also absorbs radioactive iodine, causing the gland to deteriorate.

Your thyroid gland can be surgically removed.

You'll develop hypothyroidism and need to take thyroid hormone daily if you have radioactive iodine treatment or surgery that destroys your thyroid gland.

Hypothyroidism

The inverse of hyperthyroidism is hypothyroidism. The thyroid gland is underactive, and it is incapable of producing enough hormones.

Hashimoto's thyroiditis, thyroid surgery, or radiation-induced damage are all common causes of hypothyroidism. Around 4.6 percent of people aged 12 and up in the United States are affected by it. Hypothyroidism is usually a minor problem.

Symptoms of insufficient thyroid hormone production include:

• memory problems • dry skin • increased sensitivity to cold

• constipation\s• depression

Weight gain, weakness, and a slowed heart rate are all symptoms of a slow heart rate.

• coma

Diagnosis and therapy for hypothyroidism

Thyroid hormone and TSH levels will be measured through blood tests by your doctor. Thyroid underactivity may be indicated by a high TSH level and a low thyroxine level. These levels could also mean that your pituitary gland is producing more TSH in an attempt to stimulate the thyroid gland to produce its hormone.

Taking thyroid hormone pills is the most common treatment for hypothyroidism. Because taking too much thyroid hormone can cause hyperthyroidism symptoms, it's critical to get the dose just right.

Hashimoto's thyroiditis is a condition in which the thyroid gland produces too much thyroid hormone.

Chronic lymphocytic thyroiditis, or Hashimoto's thyroiditis, is a type of thyroiditis that affects the immune system. It affects about 14 million Americans and is the most common cause of hypothyroidism in the country. It can strike anyone at any age, but middle-aged women are the most vulnerable. The thyroid gland and its ability to produce hormones are mistakenly attacked and slowly destroyed by the body's immune system.

Some people with Hashimoto's thyroiditis don't show any symptoms at all. The disease can go unnoticed for years, and the signs and symptoms are often inconspicuous. They're also non-specific, which means they can cause symptoms that are similar to those of a variety of other illnesses. • Fatigue is a symptom.

• depression

• constipation\s• mild weight gain\s• dry skin

• dry, thinning hair

• pale, puffy face

• heavy and irregular menstruation\s• intolerance to cold\s• enlarged thyroid, or goiter

Diagnosis and treatment for Hashimoto's disease

Testing the level of TSH is often the first step when screening for any type of thyroid disorder. Your doctor might order a blood test to check for increased levels of TSH as well as low levels of thyroid hormone (T3 or T4) if you're experiencing some of the above symptoms. Hashimoto's thyroiditis is an autoimmune disorder, so the blood test would also show abnormal antibodies that might be attacking the thyroid.

There's no known cure for Hashimoto's thyroiditis. Hormone-replacing medication is often used to raise thyroid hormone levels or lower TSH levels. It can also help relieve the symptoms of the disease. Surgery might be necessary to remove part or all of the thyroid gland in rare advanced cases of Hashimoto's. The disease is usually detected at an early stage and remains stable for years because it progresses slowly.

Graves' disease is a genetic condition that affects people.

Graves' disease was named for the doctor who first described it more than 150 years ago. It's the most common cause of hyperthyroidism in the United States, affecting about 1 in 200 people.

Graves' is an autoimmune disorder that occurs when the body's immune system mistakenly attacks the thyroid gland. This can cause the gland to overproduce the hormone responsible for regulating metabolism.

The disease is hereditary and may develop at any age in men or women, but it's much more common in women ages 20 to 30, according to the Department of Health and Human Services. Other risk factors include stress, pregnancy, and smoking.

When there's a high level of thyroid hormone in your bloodstream, your body's systems speed up and cause symptoms that are common to hyperthyroidism. These include:\s•anxiety\s• irritability

• fatigue

• hand tremors

• increased or irregular heartbeat

• excessive sweating\s• difficulty sleeping\s• diarrhea or frequent bowel movements

• altered menstrual cycle\s• goiter

• bulging eyes and vision problems

Diagnosing and treating Graves' disease

A simple physical exam can reveal an enlarged thyroid, enlarged bulging eyes, and signs of increased metabolism, including rapid pulse and high blood pressure. Your doctor will also order blood tests to check for high levels of T4 and low levels of TSH, both of which are signs of Graves' disease. A radioactive iodine uptake test might also be administered to measure how quickly your thyroid takes up iodine. A high uptake of iodine is consistent with Graves' disease.

There's no treatment to stop the immune system from attacking the thyroid gland and causing it to overproduce hormones. However, the symptoms of Graves' disease can be controlled in several ways, often with a combination of treatments:

• beta-blockers to control rapid heart rate, anxiety, and sweating

• antithyroid medications to prevent your thyroid from producing excessive amounts of hormone

• radioactive iodine to destroy all or part of your thyroid\s• surgery to remove your thyroid gland, a permanent option if you can't tolerate antithyroid drugs or radioactive iodine

Successful hyperthyroidism treatment usually results in hypothyroidism. You'll have to take hormone-replacement medication from that point forward. Graves' disease can lead to heart problems and brittle bones if it's left untreated.

Goiter

Goiter is a noncancerous enlargement of the thyroid gland. The most common cause of goiter worldwide is iodine deficiency in the diet. Researchers estimate that goiter affects 200 million of the 800 million people who are iodine-deficient worldwide.

Conversely, goiter is often caused by — and a symptom of — hyperthyroidism in the United States, where iodized salt provides plenty of iodine.

Goiter can affect anyone at any age, especially in areas of the world where foods rich in iodine are in short supply. However, goiters are more common after the age of 40 and in women, who are more likely to have thyroid disorders. Other risk factors include family medical history, certain medication usage, pregnancy, and radiation exposure.

There might not be any symptoms if the goiter isn't severe. The goiter may cause one or more of the following symptoms if it grows large enough, depending on the size:

• swelling or tightness in your neck\s• difficulties breathing or swallowing\s• coughing or wheezing

• hoarseness of voice

Diagnosis and therapy for goiter

Your doctor will feel your neck area and have you swallow during a routine physical exam. Blood tests will reveal the levels of thyroid hormone, TSH, and antibodies in your bloodstream. This will diagnose thyroid disorders that are often a cause of goiter. An ultrasound of the thyroid can check for swelling or nodules.

Goiter is usually treated only when it becomes severe enough to cause symptoms. You can take small doses of iodine if goiter is the result of iodine deficiency. Radioactive iodine can shrink the thyroid gland. Surgery will remove all or part of the gland. The treatments usually overlap because goiter is often a symptom of hyperthyroidism.

Goiters are often associated with highly treatable thyroid disorders, such as Graves' disease. Although goiters aren't usually a cause for concern, they can cause serious complications if they're left untreated. These complications can include difficulty breathing and swallowing.

Nodules on the thyroid

Thyroid nodules are growths that form on or in the thyroid gland. About 1 percent of men and 5 percent of women living in iodine-sufficient countries have thyroid nodules that are large enough to feel. About 50 percent of people will have nodules that are too tiny to feel.

The causes aren't always known but can include iodine deficiency and Hashimoto's thyroiditis. The nodules can be solid or fluid-filled.

Most are benign, but they can also be cancerous in a small percentage of cases. As with other thyroid-related problems, nodules are more common in women than men, and the risk in both sexes increases with age.

Most thyroid nodules don't cause any symptoms. However, if they grow large enough, they can cause swelling in your neck and lead to breathing and swallowing difficulties, pain, and goiter.

Some nodules produce thyroid hormone, causing abnormally high levels in the bloodstream. When this happens, symptoms are similar to those of hyperthyroidism and can include:\s• high pulse rate

• nervousness

• increased appetite\s• tremors

• Loss of body weight

• clammy skin

On the other hand, symptoms will be similar to hypothyroidism if the nodules are associated with Hashimoto's disease. This includes:

• fatigue

• weight gain

• hair loss\s• dry skin\s• cold intolerance

The diagnosis and treatment of thyroid nodules

Most nodules are detected during a normal physical exam. They can also be detected during an ultrasound, CT scan, or an MRI. Once a nodule is detected, other procedures — a TSH test and a thyroid scan — can check for hyperthyroidism or hypothyroidism. A fine needle aspiration biopsy is used to take a sample of cells from the nodule and determine whether the nodule is cancerous.

Benign thyroid nodules aren't life-threatening and usually don't need treatment. Typically, nothing is done to remove the nodule if it doesn't change over time. Your doctor may do another biopsy and recommend radioactive iodine to shrink the nodules if it grows.

Cancerous nodules are pretty rare — according to the National Cancer Institute, thyroid cancer affects less than 4 percent of the population. The treatment your doctor recommends will vary depending on the type of tumor. Removing the thyroid through surgery is usually the treatment of choice. Radiation therapy is sometimes used with or without surgery. Chemotherapy is often required if the cancer spreads to other parts of the body.

Common thyroid conditions in children

Children can also get thyroid conditions, including:

• hypothyroidism\s• hyperthyroidism\s• thyroid nodules

• thyroid cancer

Sometimes children are born with a thyroid problem. In other cases, surgery, disease, or treatment for another condition causes it.

Hypothyroidism

Children can get different types of hypothyroidism:

Congenital hypothyroidism occurs when the thyroid gland doesn't develop properly at birth. It affects about 1 out of every 2,500 to 3,000 babies born in the United States.

Autoimmune hypothyroidism is caused by an autoimmune disease in which the immune system attacks the thyroid gland. This type is often caused by chronic lymphocytic thyroiditis. Autoimmune hypothyroidism often appears during the teenage years, and it's more common in girls than boys.

Iatrogenic hypothyroidism happens in children who have their thyroid gland removed or destroyed — through surgery, for example.

Symptoms of hypothyroidism in children include:

• fatigue\s• weight gain

• constipation\s• intolerance to cold\s• dry, thin hair

• dry skin\s• slow heartbeat

• hoarse voice

• puffy face

• increased menstrual flow in young women Hyperthyroidism

There are multiple causes of hyperthyroidism in children:

Graves' disease is less common in children than in adults. Graves' disease often appears during the teenage years, and it affects more girls than boys.

Hyperfunctioning thyroid nodules are growths on a child's thyroid gland that produce too much thyroid hormone.

Thyroiditis is caused by inflammation in the thyroid gland that makes thyroid hormone leak out into the bloodstream.

Symptoms of hyperthyroidism in children include: • fast heart rate

• shaking • bulging eyes (in children with Graves' disease) • restlessness and irritability

• poor sleep • increased appetite • weight loss

• increased bowel movements

• intolerance to heat

• goiter

Nodules on the thyroid

Thyroid nodules are rare in children, but when they do occur, they're more likely to be cancerous. The main symptom of a thyroid nodule in a child is a lump in the neck.

Thyroid cancer

Thyroid cancer is the most common type of endocrine cancer in children, yet it's still very rare. It's diagnosed in less than 1 out of every 1 million children under age 10 each year. The

incidence is slightly higher in teens, with a rate of about 15 cases per million in 15- to 19-year- olds.

Symptoms of thyroid cancer in children include:

• a lump in the neck • swollen glands

• tight feeling in the neck • trouble breathing or swallowing • hoarse voice

Preventing thyroid dysfunction

In most cases, you can't prevent hypothyroidism or hyperthyroidism. In developing countries, hypothyroidism is often caused by iodine deficiency. However, thanks to the addition of iodine to table salt, this deficiency is rare in the United States.

Hyperthyroidism is often caused by Graves' disease, an autoimmune disease that isn't preventable. You can set off an overactive thyroid by taking too much thyroid hormone. If you're prescribed thyroid hormone, make sure to take the correct dose. In rare cases, your thyroid can become overactive if you eat too many foods that contain iodine, such as table salt, fish, and seaweed.

Though you may not be able to prevent thyroid disease, you can prevent its complications by getting diagnosed right away and following the treatment your doctor prescribes.

Hypothyroidism: The Best Diet

Hypothyroidism is a condition in which the body doesn't make enough thyroid hormones.

Thyroid hormones help control growth, cell repair, and metabolism. As a result, people with hypothyroidism may experience tiredness, hair loss, weight gain, feeling cold, and feeling down, among many other symptoms.

Hypothyroidism affects 1–2 percent of people worldwide and is 10 times more likely to affect women than men.

Foods alone won't cure hypothyroidism. However, a combination of the right nutrients and medication can help restore thyroid function and minimize your symptoms.

What is hypothyroidism

The thyroid gland is a small, butterfly-shaped gland that sits near the base of your neck. It makes and stores thyroid hormones that affect nearly every cell in your body.

When the thyroid gland receives a signal called thyroid-stimulating hormone (TSH), it releases thyroid hormones into the bloodstream. This signal is sent from the pituitary gland, a small gland found at the base of your brain, when thyroid hormone levels are low.

Occasionally, the thyroid gland doesn't release thyroid hormones, even when there is plenty of TSH. This is called primary hypothyroidism and the most common type of hypothyroidism.

Approximately 90 percent of primary hypothyroidism is caused by Hashimoto's thyroiditis, an autoimmune disease in which your immune system mistakenly attacks your thyroid gland.

Other causes of primary hypothyroidism are iodine deficiency, a genetic disorder, taking certain medications, and surgery that removes part of the thyroid.

Other times, the thyroid gland doesn't receive enough TSH. This happens when the pituitary gland is not working properly and is called secondary hypothyroidism.

Thyroid hormones are very important. They help control growth, cell repair, and metabolism — the process by which your body converts what you eat into energy.

Your metabolism affects your body temperature and at what rate you burn calories. That is why people with hypothyroidism often feel cold and fatigued and may gain weight easily.

What is the impact of hypothyroidism on metabolism?

The thyroid hormone helps control the speed of your metabolism. The faster your metabolism, the more calories your body burns at rest.

People with hypothyroidism make less thyroid hormone. This means they have a slower metabolism and burn fewer calories at rest.

Having a slow metabolism comes with several health risks. It may leave you tired, increase your blood cholesterol levels, and make it harder for you to lose weight.

If you find it difficult to maintain your weight with hypothyroidism, try doing moderate or high intensity cardio. This includes exercises like fast-paced walking, running, hiking, and rowing.

Research shows that moderate to high intensity aerobic exercise may help boost your thyroid hormone levels. In turn, this may help speed up your metabolism.

People with hypothyroidism might also benefit from increasing protein intake. Research shows that higher protein diets help increase the rate of your metabolism.

What are the most vital nutrients?

Several nutrients are important for optimal thyroid health. Iodine

Iodine is an essential mineral that is needed to make thyroid hormones. Thus, people with iodine deficiency might be at risk of hypothyroidism.

Iodine deficiency is very common and affects nearly one-third of the world's population. However, it's less common in people from developed countries like the United States, where iodized salt and iodine-rich seafood is widely available.

If you have an iodine deficiency, consider adding iodized table salt to your meals or eating more iodine-rich foods like seaweed, fish, dairy, and eggs.

Iodine supplements are unnecessary, as you can get plenty of iodine from your diet. Some studies have also shown that getting too much of this mineral may damage the thyroid gland.

Selenium Selenium helps "activate" thyroid hormones so they can be used by the body.

This essential mineral also has antioxidant benefits, which means it may protect the thyroid gland from damage by molecules called free radicals.

Adding selenium-rich foods to your diet is a great way to boost your selenium levels. This includes Brazil nuts, tuna, sardines, eggs, and legumes.

However, avoid taking a selenium supplement unless advised by a healthcare professional. Supplements provide large doses, and selenium may be toxic in large amounts.

Zinc

Like selenium, zinc helps the body "activate" thyroid hormones.

Studies also show that zinc may help the body regulate TSH, the hormone that tells the thyroid gland to release thyroid hormones.

Zinc deficiencies are rare in developed countries, as zinc is abundant in the food supply.

Nonetheless, if you have hypothyroidism, aim to eat more zinc-rich foods like oysters and other shellfish, beef, and chicken.

Which vitamins and minerals are dangerous?

Hypothyroidism patients may be harmed by a number of foods. Goitrogens

Goitrogens are substances that may disrupt the thyroid gland's natural function.

Their name comes from the word goiter, which refers to an enlargement of the thyroid gland that may arise as a result of hypothyroidism.

Goitrogens are found in a surprising number of everyday foods, including:

Tofu, tempeh, edamame, and other soy foods

Cabbage, broccoli, kale, cauliflower, spinach, and other vegetables

Sweet potatoes, cassava, peaches, strawberries, and other starchy plants Millet, pine nuts, peanuts, and other nuts and seeds

Hypothyroidism patients should avoid goitrogens in principle. However, this seems to be a problem mainly for persons who are deficient in iodine or consume a lot of goitrogens.

Cooking meals containing goitrogens may also render these chemicals inactive.

Pearl millet is an exception to the above-mentioned foods. Even if you don't have an iodine shortage, pearl millet has been proven to interfere with thyroid function in certain studies.

Things to stay away from

If you have hypothyroidism, you don't have to avoid a lot of things.

Goitrogen-containing meals, on the other hand, should be consumed in moderation and preferably prepared.

You should avoid consuming highly processed meals since they are often rich in calories. If you have hypothyroidism, this might be an issue since you may gain weight quickly.

Here's a list of foods and supplements you should stay away from:

Millet comes in a wide range of kinds.

Hot dogs, cakes, biscuits, and other highly processed meals

Supplements: Adequate selenium and iodine intakes are critical for thyroid health, but too much of either may be harmful. Only take selenium and iodine supplements if your doctor has recommended it.

Here's a list of foods that may be consumed in moderation. If ingested in significant quantities, these foods contain goitrogens or are recognized irritants:

Tofu, tempeh, edamame beans, soy milk, and other soy-based foods Peaches, pears, and strawberries, to name a few.

Coffee, green tea, and alcohol are among drinks that might aggravate your thyroid gland.

Suitable foods

If you have hypothyroidism, you may eat a variety of foods, including:

• Eggs: whole eggs are preferable since the yolk has the most iodine and selenium, while the whites are high in protein.

• Meat: any kind of meat, including lamb, beef, chicken, and so on.

• Fish: any kind of seafood, such as salmon, tuna, halibut, shrimp, and so on.

• Vegetables: all vegetables — cruciferous vegetables, particularly when prepared, are OK to consume in moderation.

• Other fruits, such as berries, bananas, oranges, tomatoes, and so on.

Rice, buckwheat, quinoa, chia seeds, and flax seeds are gluten-free grains and seeds.

• Dairy items include milk, cheese, yogurt, and other dairy products.

• Drinks: non-caffeinated beverages such as water

Hypothyroidism patients should consume a diet rich in vegetables, fruits, and lean meats. These are low in calories and filling, which may help you avoid gaining weight.

Meal plan model

For hypothyroidism, here is a 7-day diet plan.

It includes a good quantity of protein, a low to moderate amount of carbohydrates, and may help you lose weight.

Take your thyroid medicine at least 1–2 hours before your first meal, or as directed by your healthcare provider. Fiber, calcium, and iron may prevent your body from effectively absorbing thyroid medicine.

Monday

• Eggs on toast for breakfast

• Chicken salad with 2–3 Brazil nuts for lunch; stir-fried chicken and veggies with rice for dinner Tuesday

• Oatmeal with 1/4 cup (31 grams) fruit for breakfast

• Lunch: grilled salmon salad • Dinner: lemon, thyme, and black pepper baked fish with steamed veggies Wednesday

• Eggs on toast for breakfast

• Dinner leftovers for lunch

• Dinner: shrimp skewers with quinoa salad Thursday • Breakfast: overnight chia pudding with sliced fruits of your choice — 2 tbsp. (28 grams) chia seeds, 1 cup (240 mL) Greek yogurt, 1/2 tsp. vanilla extract, and sliced fruits of your choice Allow to rest overnight in a dish or Mason jar.

• Lunch: dinner leftovers • Dinner: roast lamb with sautéed veggies • Breakfast on Friday: a banana-berry smoothie

• Chicken salad sandwich for lunch

• Dinner: pork fajitas on corn tortillas with sliced lean meat, bell peppers, and salsa Saturday

• Frittata with eggs, mushrooms, and zucchini for breakfast

• Lunch: tuna and boiled egg salad; dinner: tomato paste, olives, and feta cheese on handmade Mediterranean pizza • Breakfast on Sunday: omelet with a variety of veggies

• Quinoa salad with green veggies and almonds for lunch

• Steak grilled with a side salad for dinner

Weight-loss recommendations

Due to a slowed metabolism, hypothyroidism makes it extremely simple to acquire weight. Here are some suggestions to help you maintain a healthy body weight:

• Make sure you get enough of rest. Every night, try to obtain 7–8 hours of sleep. Sleep deprivation has been related to weight increase, particularly around the abdomen.

• Make mindful eating a habit. Mindful eating, which is paying attention to what you're eating, why you're eating, and how quickly you're eating, may aid in the development of a healthier relationship with food. It has also been shown in studies to aid weight loss.

• Try meditating or doing yoga. De-stressing and improving your general health may be achieved via yoga and meditation. They may also help you control your weight, according to research.

•

Try eating a low- to moderate-carbohydrate diet. It is quite effective to lose weight by eating a low to moderate quantity of carbohydrates. However, a ketogenic diet should be avoided since eating too little carbohydrates might cause your thyroid hormone levels to drop.

Recipes

Sheet Pan Eggs with Veggies and Parmesan • 6 Servings • 5 Minute Prep Time • 15 Minute Cook Time Ingredients: 12 large whisked eggs

- Seasoning (salt and pepper)

- 1 tiny sliced red pepper • 1 small minced yellow onion

- 1 cup mushrooms, diced

- 1 cup zucchini, diced

- 1 cup parmesan cheese (freshly grated) • Preheat the oven to 350 degrees F and coat a rimmed baking sheet with cooking spray.

- In a mixing bowl, whisk the eggs with salt and pepper until foamy.

- Combine the peppers, onions, mushrooms, and zucchini in a large mixing bowl.

- Pour the batter onto the baking sheet and spread it out evenly.

- Top with parmesan cheese and bake for 12–15 minutes, or until the egg is set.

-

Allow to cool somewhat before serving in squares.

215 calories, 14 grams of fat, 18.5 grams of protein, 5 grams of carbohydrates, 1 gram of fiber, and 4 grams of net carbohydrates

4 Servings Grilled Pesto Salmon with Asparagus

• 5 minute prep time

• Preparation Time: 15 minutes • 4 boneless salmon fillets (6 ounces) • Salt and pepper • 1 bunch asparagus, ends trimmed

• 2 tblsp. extra virgin olive oil

• 14 cup pesto (basil) • Oil the grates of a grill and preheat it to high heat.

•

Spray the salmon with cooking spray after seasoning it with salt and pepper.

• Cook the salmon for 4 to 5 minutes on each side, or until done.

• Toss the asparagus with the oil and cook for approximately 10 minutes, or until tender.

• Drizzle the pesto over the salmon and serve with asparagus on the side.

300 calories, 17.5 grams of fat, 34.5 grams of protein, 2.5 grams of carbohydrates, 1.5 grams of fiber, and 1 gram of net carbohydrates

4 servings of Cheddar-Stuffed Zucchini Burgers

• Time to prepare: 10 minutes

• Preparation Time: 15 minutes Ingredients: 1 pound of beef (80% lean) and 2 big eggs

• a quarter cup of almond flour

• Salt and pepper • 1 cup shredded cheddar cheese

• 2 tblsp. extra virgin olive oil

• 1 big halved and sliced zucchini • In a mixing dish, combine the meat, egg, almond flour, cheese, salt, and pepper.

•

Mix well, then divide into four equal-sized patties.

• In a large skillet, heat the oil over medium-high heat.

• Cook for 5 minutes, or until the burger patties are browned.

•

Toss the zucchini in the pan with the patties to coat it with oil.

• Season the zucchini with salt and pepper and simmer for 5 minutes, stirring periodically.

•

Serve the burgers with a side of zucchini and your preferred toppings.

470 calories, 29.5 grams of fat, 47 grams of protein, 4.5 grams of carbohydrates, 1.5 grams of fiber, and 3 grams of net carbohydrates

4 Servings Chicken Cordon Bleu with Cauliflower

• Time to prepare: 10 minutes

• Preparation Time: 45 minutes • 4 boneless chicken breast halves (about 12 oz.) • 4 slices deli ham • 4 slices Swiss cheese

• 1 big egg, whisked thoroughly

• Pork rinds, 2 oz.

12 teaspoon garlic powder • 14 cup almond flour • 14 cup grated parmesan cheese

• Seasoning (salt and pepper)

• 2 cups florets de cauliflower • Preheat the oven to 350 degrees Fahrenheit and line a baking sheet with foil.

• Place the chicken breast halves between parchment paper and pound them flat.

• Arrange the pieces on a serving platter and top with sliced ham and cheese.

• Wrap the chicken around the fillings before dipping it in the beaten egg.

• Pulse the pork rinds, almond flour, parmesan, garlic powder, salt, and pepper into small crumbs in a food processor.

•

Place the chicken rolls on the baking sheet after rolling them in the pork rind mixture.

• Toss the cauliflower with the melted butter before transferring it to the baking sheet.

• Bake for 45 minutes, or until chicken is well done.

420 calories, 23.5 grams of fat, 45 grams of protein, 7 grams of carbohydrates, 2.5 grams of fiber, and 4.5 grams of net carbohydrates

Tuna with Sesame Crusted Green Beans • 4 Servings

• 15-minute prep time

• Preparation Time: 5 minutes 14 cup white sesame seeds, plus 14 cup black sesame seeds

• 4 ahi tuna steaks (6 oz.)

• 1 tablespoon olive oil • salt and pepper

• 2 cups green beans • 1 tablespoon coconut oil • In a shallow plate, mix together the two varieties of sesame seeds.

•

Using salt and pepper, season the tuna.

• In a pan over high heat, dredge the tuna in the sesame seed mixture, then add it to the olive oil.

• Cook for 1 to 2 minutes until sear marks appear on the surface, then flip and sear the other side.

• Remove the tuna from the pan and set aside to rest while the skillet is reheated with the coconut oil.

• Fry the green beans for 5 minutes in the oil before serving with sliced tuna.

380 calories, 19 grams of fat, 44.5 grams of protein, 8 grams of carbohydrates, 3 grams of fiber, and 5 grams of net carbohydrates

4 Servings Rosemary Roasted Pork with Cauliflower

• Time to prepare: 10 minutes • Time to cook: 20 minutes 12 pound boneless pork tenderloin 1 tablespoon coconut oil 1 tablespoon fresh chopped rosemary

• 1 tablespoon olive oil • salt and pepper

• 2 cups florets de cauliflower • Rub the pork with coconut oil before seasoning it with rosemary, salt, and pepper.

• In a large pan, heat the olive oil over medium-high heat.

• Cook for 2 to 3 minutes on each side, until the pork is browned.

• Arrange the cauliflower in a circle around the meat in the pan.

• Reduce the heat to low, cover the pan, and simmer for 8 to 10 minutes, or until the pork is well cooked.

• Cut the pork into slices and serve with the cauliflower.

300 calories, 15.5 grams of fat, 37 grams of protein, 3 grams of carbohydrates, 1.5 grams of fiber, and 1.5 grams of net carbohydrates

Ingredients for a Quick Mexican Soup

• 1 pound boneless skinless chicken thighs, cut into 3/4-inch pieces • 1 tablespoon taco seasoning with reduced sodium

• 1 carton (32 ounces) reduced-sodium chicken broth • 1 cup frozen corn • 1 cup salsa

Directions

• Heat the oil in a big saucepan over high heat. Cook for 6-8 minutes, stirring occasionally, until the chicken is no longer pink. • Add additional ingredients and bring to a boil, stirring in taco seasoning. Reduce heat to low and continue to cook for 5 minutes, uncovered, to enable flavors to meld. Before serving, skim off the fat.

Ingredients for Roasted Tomato Soup with Basil

- 3 1/2 pound tomatoes, halved (about 11 medium)

2 garlic cloves, peeled and halved • 1 small onion, quartered

1 teaspoon salt • 2 tablespoons olive oil • 2 tablespoons fresh thyme leaves

12 fresh basil leaves, 1/4 teaspoon pepper

- Thinly sliced fresh basil and salad croutons, if desired Directions

- Heat the oven to 400 degrees Fahrenheit. In a greased 15x10x1-inch baking pan, combine tomatoes, onion, and garlic; drizzle with olive oil. Toss to coat with thyme, salt, and pepper. Roast for 25-30 minutes, stirring once during the cooking process, until the vegetables are tender. Allow to cool a bit.

-

In a blender, blend the tomato mixture and basil leaves until smooth, in batches. Fill a large saucepan halfway with water and bring to a boil. Croutons and sliced basil can be added if desired.

Ingredients for Soup with Turkey Sausage, Butternut Squash, and Kale

• 1 medium butternut squash (about 3 pounds), peeled and cubed • 2 cartons Italian turkey sausage links (19-1/2 ounces) with casings removed chicken broth with low sodium

• 1/2 cup shaved Parmesan cheese • 1 bunch kale, trimmed and coarsely chopped (roughly 16 cups) Directions

• Cook sausage in a stockpot over medium heat, breaking it up into crumbles, until it's no longer pink, about 8 to 10 minutes.

• Bring to a boil the squash and broth. Stir in the kale in small batches, allowing it to wilt slightly between each addition. Raise the temperature to high and bring the water back to a boil. Reduce to a low heat and cook, covered, for 15-20 minutes, or until vegetables are tender. Serve with a dollop of sour cream on top.

Facts on Nutrition

1 cup contains 163 calories, 5 grams of fat (2 grams of saturated fat), 23 milligrams of cholesterol, 838 milligrams of sodium, 20 grams of carbohydrates (5 grams of sugar, 5 grams of fiber), and 13 grams of protein.

Dessert Cups in Chocolate

12 cups yielded 15-Minute Preparation 2 minutes to prepare 40 minutes inactive time

These elegant little chocolate cups elevate creamy keto desserts in an instant. Fill them with Whipped Cream and a berry on top, or just fill them with Whipped Cream. They're the ideal size for a small bite-size dessert.

Ingredients

• 2 oz. dark chocolate, sugar-free, chopped

• 14 oz cacao butter (or 112 oz coconut oil) Directions

• In a mini muffin pan, line 12 liners with silicone or parchment paper.

In a microwave-safe bowl, combine the chocolate and cacao butter. Microwave in 30-second increments on high power, stirring after each, until melted and smooth. In a heatproof bowl set over a pan of barely simmering water, melt the chocolate and cacao butter together.

• Using the back of a spoon, evenly coat the bottom and sides of each mini muffin liner with melted chocolate. There should be enough chocolate left over.

• Place the cups in the refrigerator for 10 minutes, then recoat the sides and cover any thin areas with the remaining chocolate. Refrigerate for 30 minutes or until firm.

• Remove the muffin liners by gently peeling them away.

Directions for storage: These cups will keep in the fridge for several weeks, ready to use whenever you want.

Tips: For these cups, I prefer to use silicone liners because they peel off easily. With my thumb on the inside and my forefinger on the outside, I pinch the bottom half of the cup. With my other hand, I carefully peel the liner away. You can also make regular muffin-size cups, but you'll only get four, which means the carb count per serving will be slightly higher.

About 212 cups of chocolate buttercream frosting 10 minute prep time — minutes to cook Yes, I know, cream cheese shouldn't be used in buttercream. But here's the thing: traditional frostings call for a ridiculous amount of powdered sugar to achieve the right consistency. I simply no longer enjoy sweet foods, and powdered sugar substitutes are prohibitively expensive. Without adding 2 or 3 cups of powdered sweetener, a small amount of cream cheese gives this frosting structure.

• 1 tablespoon coconut oil • 2 ounces chopped unsweetened chocolate

12 cup unsalted butter (1 stick), softened

• 2 cup powdered erythritol-based sweetener • 3 ounces softened cream cheese (14% cup plus 2 tablespoons)

• cocoa powder (2 tbsp.)

• 12 teaspoon extract de vanille

• 14–12 cup room-temperature heavy whipping cream • A powdered bulk sweetener is the best option here because it provides structure for a proper frosting. Directions

• Melt the chocolate with the coconut oil in a medium microwave-safe bowl. Microwave on high for 30 seconds, stirring after each increment, until smooth and melted. In a heatproof bowl set over a pan of barely simmering water, melt the chocolate and coconut oil. Allow to cool to room temperature before serving.

• Cream the butter and cream cheese together in a large mixing bowl until completely smooth. Combine the sweetener and cocoa powder in a mixing bowl and beat until smooth.

• Mix in the melted chocolate and vanilla extract until well combined. At this point, the mixture will be thick.

•

Add a few tablespoons of cream at a time until you reach a spreadable consistency.

Spread this frosting on top of the One-Bowl Brownies for an extra-special chocolate treat. With the Slice-and-Bake Vanilla Wafers, you can also make fun little sandwich cookies. Make one of the low-carb cake mixes from Swerve or Good Dee's and top it with this delicious buttercream if you need a quick birthday cake.

This buttercream can be kept in the fridge for up to a week, but it has the best consistency and spreadability when made fresh.

This frosting recipe serves 12 cupcakes or one 8-inch single layer cake.

Chocolate-hazelnut spread made from scratch

3 cup (yield) 10 minute prep time — minutes to cook I wish you could see how frequently I whip up this Nutella-style spread. It's a big hit with my kids, and they eat it almost every morning with their low-carb muffins. If I want any, I have to fend off the kids or hide the jar!

Ingredients

• toasted and husked 34 cup hazelnuts

• melted coconut oil (about 2 to 3 tablespoons)

12 teaspoon vanilla extract • 2 tablespoons cocoa powder • 2 tablespoons powdered erythritol-based sweetener salt (a pinch) Options for sweetener:

This spread thickens with a powdered bulk sweetener, but any sweetener will suffice. Instructions • Finely grind the hazelnuts in a food processor or high-powered blender until they clump together.

• Blend in 2 tablespoons coconut oil until a smooth butter forms. Blend together the cocoa powder, sweetener, vanilla extract, and salt until smooth. It's best if the mixture is a little runny. Add the last tablespoon of oil if it's too thick.

Directions for storage: This spread will keep in the fridge for a long time because it contains no perishable ingredients. You won't be able to keep it for very long, though! It will firm up in the fridge, but at room temperature, it will revert to a more liquid-like state.

Trader Joe's sells pre-roasted, husked, unsalted hazelnuts if you live near one. I buy four bags at a time, which is a total lifesaver. Other brands can also be found online. If you must roast and husk your own hazelnuts, I find that rubbing the toasted nuts between my fingers until most of the skin falls off is the most effective method. Don't worry about getting them completely free of husks. You can substitute another oil for the coconut oil, but I find that at room temperature, coconut oil makes it less liquidy than a liquid oil.

Your food processor or blender's ability to make a smooth chocolate hazelnut spread is largely determined by its quality.

Sauce with Caramel

1 cup (approximate) 5 minutes to prepare 10 minutes to prepare I worked hard to create a low-carb caramel sauce that I was proud of. This one hits all the right notes for me in terms of flavor, color, consistency, and nutritional value.

Ingredients

• 14 cup unsalted butter (12 stick) • 14 cup plus 2 tablespoons granulated erythritol sweetener

12 cup heavy whipping cream • 14 teaspoon xanthan gum • 2 teaspoons yacón syrup (optional)

• 1 tablespoon water • 14 teaspoon kosher or medium-grind sea salt • Granulated erythritol or a granulated erythritol-based blend is the only sugar substitute that caramelizes, so it's your only choice for this recipe.

Directions

• Melt the butter, sweetener, and yacón syrup, if using, in a medium saucepan over medium heat, stirring constantly until the sweetener dissolves. Bring to a boil, then reduce heat to low and continue to cook for 3 to 5 minutes, or until the color darkens.

• Turn off the heat and stir in the cream. There will be a lot of bubbling in the mixture. Whisk vigorously to incorporate the xanthan gum. After that, sprinkle the salt on top.

• Boil for another minute on medium heat. Allow to cool to room temperature before stirring in the water.

Directions for storage: This sauce will keep for about a week in the fridge. (I've had mine for a couple of weeks now.) To make it pourable again, simply reheat it gently in the microwave or in a saucepan.

You can omit the yacón syrup if you prefer, but it will give your sauce a richer caramel flavor and color. Blackstrap molasses can also be substituted. Each serving of yacón syrup and blackstrap molasses contains only about 1 gram of carbs.

Sprinkled Coconut

1 tablespoon of final product 1 minute of preparation — minutes to cook My friends at Keto Kookie informed me that using colored shredded coconut as sprinkles is a brilliant

idea. I had to give it a shot, and I must say, it's a brilliant concept. It adds a touch of holiday cheer to keto desserts.

1 tablespoon shredded unsweetened coconut • natural food coloring in desired color

Storage advice: As long as your coconut is in good shape, these sprinkles will last almost indefinitely. In my baking cupboard, I keep a small jar of the mixed colors, ready to use whenever I need some fun sprinkles!

Directions

• In a small mixing bowl, combine the shredded coconut and a drop or two of food coloring. • Allow to dry until ready to use if using powdered food coloring. For any other colors of sprinkles, repeat with more coconut.

Whipping Cream of Coconut

Yield: About 1 cup (¼ cup per serving) Prep Time: 8 minutes, plus time to chill milk, bowl, and beaters — minutes to cook Coconut whipped cream is a fabulous dairy-free alternative to the real thing. It rocks its own special coconut flavor, and I like to bring that out even more by adding a little coconut extract. The trick is to chill the can of coconut milk for at least eight hours, if not more; it won't whip properly when it's warm.

Ingredients

• 1 (13.5-ounce) can full-fat coconut milk, chilled overnight\s• 2 tablespoons powdered erythritol-based sweetener

• ½ teaspoon coconut or vanilla extract Sweetener options:\s• Any sweetener will do here. Directions

• Chill a mixing bowl and beaters in the fridge for at least 10 to 15 minutes.

• Skim the solid portion (or coconut cream) of the coconut milk from the top of the can into the chilled mixing bowl. Discard the thinner coconut water or reserve it for another use. Beat the coconut cream with an electric mixer until it is smooth and light and holds soft peaks.

• Add the sweetener and coconut extract and beat until just combined. Refrigerate until ready to use. The whipped cream will firm up in the refrigerator, so be sure to let it warm a bit on the counter before serving.

Directions for storage: Keep refrigerated until ready to use. This whipped cream will keep for as long as your coconut milk is good, up to 2 weeks.

Sheet Pan Eggs With Veggies And Parmesan\s• Servings: 6

• 5 minutes to prepare

• 15-minute cook time Ingredients:\s• 12 large eggs, whisked\s• Salt and pepper\s• 1 small red pepper, diced

• 1 small yellow onion, chopped

• 1 c. mushrooms (diced)

• 1 cup diced zucchini\s• 1 cup freshly grated parmesan cheese • Preheat the oven to 350°F and lightly grease a rimmed baking sheet.

• In a mixing bowl, whisk the eggs until frothy, seasoning with salt and pepper.

• In a large mixing bowl, combine the peppers, onions, mushrooms, and zucchini.

•

Pour the mixture in the baking sheet and spread into an even layer.

•

Sprinkle with parmesan and bake for 12 to 15 minutes until the egg is set.

• Let cool slightly, then cut into squares to serve.

215 calories, 14 grams of fat, 18.5 grams of protein, 5 grams of carbohydrates, 1 gram of fiber, and 4 grams of net carbohydrates.

Salmon with Asparagus and Pesto Grilled • 4 Servings

• 5 minutes to prepare

• 15-minute cook time 4 (6-ounce) boneless salmon fillets • Salt and pepper • 1 bunch trimmed asparagus

2 tbsp. extra virgin olive oil

14 cup pesto (basil) • Oil the grill grates and preheat the grill to high heat.

•

Cooking spray the salmon after seasoning it with salt and pepper.

• Cook the salmon for 4 to 5 minutes on each side, or until fully cooked.

• Brush the asparagus with oil and grill for about 10 minutes, or until tender.

• Drizzle the pesto on top of the salmon and serve with asparagus.

300 calories, 17.5 grams of fat, 34.5 grams of protein, 2.5 grams of carbohydrate, 1.5 grams of fiber, and 1 gram of net carbohydrate

Burgers with Zucchini and Cheddar Stuffing • 4 Servings

• 10 minute prep time

• 15-minute cook time • 1 pound 80 percent lean ground beef • 2 large eggs

• a quarter-cup of almond flour

• 1 cup shredded cheddar cheese

• Season to taste with salt and pepper.

2 tbsp. extra virgin olive oil

• 1 halved and sliced large zucchini • In a large mixing bowl, whisk together the beef, egg, almond flour, cheese, salt, and pepper.

•

Combine all ingredients in a mixing bowl, then form four equal-sized patties.

• In a large skillet, heat the oil on medium-high.

• Cook for 5 minutes, or until the burger patties are golden brown.

•

Toss the zucchini in the skillet with the patties to coat it in oil before flipping them.

• Season with salt and pepper, then cook, stirring occasionally, for 5 minutes.

•

Serve the burgers with the zucchini on the side and your favorite toppings.

470 calories, 29.5 grams of fat, 47 grams of protein, 4.5 grams of carbohydrates, 1.5 grams of fiber, and 3 grams of net carbohydrates.

Cauliflower and Chicken Cordon Bleu • 4 Servings

• 10 minute prep time

• 45-minute cook time • 4 boneless chicken breast halves (approximately 12 ounces) • 4 slices deli ham

• 1 well-beaten large egg

Pork rinds, 2 oz.

• 12 teaspoon garlic powder • 14 cup almond flour • 14 cup grated parmesan cheese

• Season to taste with salt and pepper.

2 c. florets de cauliflower • Preheat oven to 350 degrees Fahrenheit and line a baking sheet with foil.

• Place the chicken breast halves on parchment paper and pound flat.

• Arrange the pieces on a serving platter and top with ham slices and cheese.

• Wrap the chicken around the fillings and dip it into the beaten egg.

• In a food processor, pulse together the pork rinds, almond flour, parmesan, garlic powder, salt, and pepper until fine crumbs form.

•

Place the chicken rolls on a baking sheet after rolling them in the pork rind mixture.

• Toss the cauliflower with the melted butter before putting it on the baking sheet.

• Bake the chicken for 45 minutes, or until it is fully cooked.

420 calories, 23.5 grams of fat, 45 grams of protein, 7 grams of carbohydrates, 2.5 grams of fiber, and 4.5 grams of net carbohydrates.

Green Beans with Sesame Crusted Tuna • 4 Servings

• 15-Minute Preparation

• 5 minutes to prepare 14 cup white sesame seeds • 14 cup black sesame seeds

Ingredients

4 ahi tuna steaks (6 ounces)

1 tablespoon olive oil • salt and pepper

2 cups green beans and 1 tablespoon coconut oil • In a shallow dish, mix together the two kinds of sesame seeds.

•

Add salt and pepper to the tuna.

• In a skillet over high heat, dredge the tuna in the sesame seed mixture.

• Cook for 1–2 minutes until seared on one side, then flip and sear on the other.

• Remove the tuna from the skillet and set aside to rest while the skillet is reheated with coconut oil.

• Cook the green beans for 5 minutes in the oil before serving with sliced tuna.

380 calories, 19 grams of fat, 44.5 grams of protein, 8 grams of carbohydrate, 3 grams of fiber, and 5 grams of net carbohydrate

4 Servings Rosemary Roasted Pork and Cauliflower

• 10 minutes to prepare • 20 minutes to cook • 12 pound boneless pork tenderloin • 1 tablespoon coconut oil • 1 tablespoon fresh rosemary

1 tablespoon olive oil • salt and pepper

2 c. florets de cauliflower • Season the pork with rosemary, salt, and pepper after rubbing it with coconut oil.

• In a large pan over medium-high heat, heat the olive oil.

• Cook for 2 to 3 minutes on each side, or until the pork is browned.

• Toss the cauliflower around the meat in the skillet.

• Reduce the heat to low, cover the pan, and simmer for 8 to 10 minutes, or until the pork is fully cooked.

• Cut the pork into slices and serve it beside the cauliflower.

300 calories, 15.5 grams of fat, 37 grams of protein, 3 grams of carbohydrates, 1.5 grams of fiber, and 1.5 grams of net carbohydrates.

Ingredients in a Quick Mexican Soup

• 1 pound boneless, skinless chicken thighs, cut into 3/4-inch pieces • 1 tablespoon taco seasoning with reduced sodium

• 1 carton (32 ounces) reduced-sodium chicken broth • 1 cup frozen corn • 1 cup salsa

Directions

• Heat the oil in a big saucepan over high heat. Cook for 6-8 minutes, stirring occasionally, until the chicken is no longer pink. • Add additional ingredients and bring to a boil, stirring in taco seasoning. Reduce heat to low and continue to cook for 5 minutes, uncovered, to enable flavors to meld. Before serving, skim off the fat.

Ingredients for Roasted Tomato Soup with Basil

• 3 1/2 pound tomatoes, halved (about 11 medium)

2 garlic cloves, peeled and halved • 1 small onion, quartered

1 teaspoon salt • 2 tablespoons olive oil • 2 tablespoons fresh thyme leaves

12 fresh basil leaves, 1/4 teaspoon pepper

• Thinly sliced fresh basil and salad croutons, if desired Directions

• Heat the oven to 400 degrees Fahrenheit. In a greased 15x10x1-inch baking pan, combine tomatoes, onion, and garlic; sprinkle with olive oil. Toss to coat with thyme, salt, and pepper. Roast for 25-30 minutes, tossing once throughout the cooking process, until the vegetables are soft. Allow to cool a little.

•

In a blender, puree the tomato mixture and basil leaves until smooth, in stages. Fill a big saucepan halfway with water and bring to a boil. Croutons and chopped basil may be added if desired.

Ingredients for a Delicious Italian Vegetable Soup

• 1 medium onion, sliced • 1-1/2 cups water • 1 pound bulk Italian sausage

• 1 can (15 ounces) washed and drained garbanzo beans or chickpeas • 1 can (14-1/2 ounces) chopped tomatoes, undrained

• 1 beef broth can (14 1/2 ounces)

• 2 medium zucchini slices, 1/4-inch thick

• 1/2 teaspoon basil (dried)

• Grated Parmesan cheese • Cook sausage and onion in a large skillet over medium heat until meat is no longer pink; drain. In a large mixing bowl, combine the water, beans, tomatoes, broth, zucchini, and basil.

• Bring the water to a boil. Reduce the heat to low and cook for 5 minutes, or until the zucchini is soft. Serve with cheese as a garnish.

Facts on Nutrition

1 cup has 173 calories, 9 grams of fat (3 grams of saturated fat), 23 milligrams of cholesterol, 620 milligrams of sodium, 14 grams of carbohydrate (5 grams of sugar, 3 grams of fiber), and 10 grams of protein.

Ingredients for Soup with Turkey Sausage, Butternut Squash, and Kale

• 1 medium butternut squash (approximately 3 pounds), peeled and diced • 2 cartons Italian turkey sausage links (19-1/2 ounces) with casings removed (32 ounces each) chicken broth with low sodium

• 1/2 cup shaved Parmesan cheese • 1 bunch kale, cut and finely chopped (about 16 cups) Directions

• Cook sausage in a stockpot over medium heat, breaking it up into crumbles, until it's no longer pink, about 8 to 10 minutes.

• Bring to a boil the squash and broth. Stir in the kale in small batches, letting it to wilt slightly between each addition. Raise the temperature to high and bring the water back to a boil. Reduce to a low heat and cook, covered, for 15-20 minutes, or until veggies are soft. Serve with a dollop of sour cream on top.

Facts on Nutrition

1 cup has 163 calories, 5 grams of fat (2 grams of saturated fat), 23 milligrams of cholesterol, 838 milligrams of sodium, 20 grams of carbohydrates (5 grams of sugars, 5 grams of fiber), and 13 grams of protein.

Ingredients for Tuscan Cauliflower Soup

• 4 cups fresh cauliflowerets (approximately 14 ounces) • 2 cans reduced-sodium chicken broth (14-1/2 ounces each) • 2 cups water

• 2 chopped garlic cloves • 1 pound Italian sausage in bulk • 1 cup sliced fresh mushrooms

• 1/4 teaspoon pepper • 1 cup thick whipped cream

- 1/2 pound cooked and crumbled bacon strips Directions

- Bring cauliflower, broth, water, and garlic to a boil in a large pot. Simmer, uncovered, for 12-15 minutes, or until cauliflower is soft.

- Meanwhile, in a large pan, sauté sausage and mushrooms over medium heat, breaking up sausage into pieces, until sausage is no longer pink, 6-8 minutes. Drain on paper towels after removing with a slotted spoon.

- Return the cauliflower mixture to a boil with the meat and mushrooms. Reduce heat to low and cook for 5 minutes, uncovered. Heat through the cream and pepper. Serve with bacon on the side.

Facts on Nutrition

1 and a half cups: 358 calories, 30 grams of fat (14 grams of saturated fat), 91 milligrams of cholesterol, 941 milligrams of sodium, 7 grams of carbohydrate (4 grams of sugar, 1 gram of fiber), 17 grams of protein

Ingredients for Shrimp & Cod Stew in Tomato-Saffron Broth

- 2 tablespoons olive oil • 1 big diced onion • 3 minced garlic cloves

• 2 bay leaves • 1 tablespoon minced fresh or 1 teaspoon dried thyme • 1/4 teaspoon saffron threads or 1 teaspoon crushed turmeric

• 2 cans (each 14 1/2 ounces) chopped tomatoes with no salt added

• 1 pound fillet of fish, cut into 1 inch cubes

• 2 cups water • 1 can (14-1/2 ounces) vegetable broth • 1 pound uncooked big shrimp, peeled and deveined

• 1 cup corn (whole kernel)

• a quarter teaspoon of pepper

• Optional lemon wedges • 1 package (6 ounces) fresh baby spinach Directions

• Heat the oil in a 6-quart stockpot over medium heat. Cook, stirring constantly, until the onion is soft. Garlic, thyme, saffron, and bay leaves should be added now. 1 minute more cooking and stirring • Bring the tomatoes, shrimp, water, broth, corn, and pepper to a boil. Reduce heat to low and cook, uncovered, for 8-10 minutes, or until shrimp are pink and fish flakes easily with a fork, stirring occasionally. Add spinach during the final 2-3 minutes of cooking. Bay leaves should be discarded. Serve with lemon wedges if preferred.

Facts on Nutrition

250 calories per 1-1/2 cup, 6 grams of fat (1 gram saturated fat), 121 milligrams of cholesterol, 1005 milligrams of sodium, 18 grams of carbohydrate (7 grams sugars, 3 grams fiber), and 27 grams of protein

Ingredients for Cheesy Broccoli Soup in a Bread Bowl

- 1/4 cup cubed butter

- 1/2 cup chopped onion • 2 minced garlic cloves

- 4 cups fresh broccoli florets (about 8 ounces) • 1 big carrot, coarsely chopped

- 2 bay leaves • 2 cups half-and-half cream

- 1/4 teaspoon powdered nutmeg • 1/2 teaspoon salt • 1/4 teaspoon pepper

- 1/4 cup cornstarch • 1/4 cup chicken stock or extra water

- 2 1/2 cups shredded cheddar cheese • 6 tiny round bread loaves (each weighing around 8 ounces)

- Toppings (optional): Cooked bacon crumbles, more shredded cheddar cheese, nutmeg, and pepper

Directions

- Melt butter in a 6-quart stockpot over medium heat and sauté onion and garlic until soft, about 6-8 minutes. Bring to a boil with the broccoli, carrot, stock, cream, and spices. Cook, uncovered, for 10-12 minutes, or until veggies are soft.

- Whisk together the cornstarch and water until smooth, then incorporate it into the soup. Bring to a boil, stirring regularly; simmer and stir for 1-2 minutes, or until thickened. Take out the bay leaves. Stir in the cheese until it is completely melted.

- To make bread bowls, take a slice from the top of each loaf and hollow out the bottoms, leaving 1/4-inch thick shells (save removed bread for another use). Just before serving, add the soup.

• Toppings may be added to the soup if desired. • These make a filling supper on their own, but they're also great as an appetizer. Smaller, more durable breads, such firm rolls, are a wonderful option.

• Maintain a calm demeanor. Allowing the soup to cool somewhat before adding cheese helps to avoid gritty cheese sauces. Stir in a little amount at a time until it melts completely.

Facts on Nutrition

422 calories, 32 grams of fat (19 grams of saturated fat), 107 milligrams of cholesterol, 904 milligrams of sodium, 15 grams of carbohydrate (5 grams of carbohydrates, 2 grams of fiber), 17 grams of protein per cup (calculated without the bread bowl).

Ingredients for Chocolate Fudge Ripple

• 1 cup thick coconut milk (8 fl oz) OR heavy cream Sugar-free marshmallows, 5 oz. / 140g

• 1 oz. (30 g) unsweetened cocoa powder

• Chopped 4 oz. / 110g 100% cocoa solids chocolate (unsweetened)

• 12 tsp vanilla extract • 2 TBSP vegetable glycerin • In a saucepan over medium heat, warm the thick coconut milk or cream. In the same pan, add the sugar-free marshmallows and stir continually until they are fully melted. • Remove the pan from the heat and stir in the cocoa powder until it is thoroughly incorporated into the marshmallow mixture. • Remove the pan from the heat and stir in the chopped chocolate. Stir constantly until all of the chocolate has melted. Stir in the glycerin and vanilla extract well.

• Transfer to a glass bowl or dish to cool fully. Cover and store in the fridge after it's cooled.

Note

This ripple is rather large. And it's dark, glossy, chocolatey, and totally, utterly magnificent. Once you've created the sugar-free marshmallows, it's very simple to put together. It is incredibly stable, freezing no harder than it is when thoroughly cooled. I sobbed with joy as I finished this final version. If only you knew the difficulties I had in making you a delicious KETO Chocolate Fudge Ripple for your ice cream. At -18°C, it remains soft, gooey, and delectable. You're totally deserving of it. If it becomes dull or stiff after being made ahead of time, just reheat gently and chill again. You can also use this sauce to drizzle over whatever you want to drizzle chocolate fudge sauce over. It keeps for weeks in the fridge, so make a large batch and have some on hand for any Chocolate Fudge Sauce emergencies. I promise you'll use this recipe often.

Ingredients for Bacon Ripple

- 12 oz. / 335g bacon

- 3 oz. / 85g xylitol (NO substitutes!)

- 2 TBSP apple cider vinegar

- 1 ½ cups / 12 fl oz. water\s• ½ tsp. liquid smoke\s• 1 ½ TBSP maple extract

- 1 ½ TBSP vegetable glycerin\s• 1 TBSP avocado oil

- ½ tsp. guar gum Directions\s• Chop the bacon into small pieces – think how big you want in a bite of ice cream – and sauté over a medium heat in a frying pan until cooked, but not crispy.

• Carefully drain off the liquid fat, and then tip the bacon onto several sheets of kitchen paper to absorb any excess grease.

• Return the bacon pieces to the pan and add the xylitol, apple cider vinegar, water, liquid smoke, maple extract and vegetable glycerin. Stir well and bring to the boil over a medium heat.

• Pour the avocado oil into a small dish and add the guar gum. Stir well until the guar gum is completely mixed in.

•

Pour the guar mixture into the hot bacon sauce and stir well until the sauce is thickened.

•

Remove from the heat and allow to cool. Pour into an airtight container and store in the fridge until you want to ripple it into the freshly churned.

Sour Cherry Chunks\sIngredients

• 8 oz. / 225g sour cherries (canned), very well drained

• 1 TBSP xylitol\s• 1 TBSP vegetable glycerin Directions

• Tip the well-drained cherries onto several sheets of kitchen paper and blot them to remove as much excess juice as possible.\s•

Place the cherries in a small pan with the xylitol and glycerin, stir well, and heat gently until just warm. Remove from the heat, stir well, and leave the cherries to soak until cold. Pour the cherries into an airtight container and store in the fridge.\s• An hour before you are ready to layer the cherries into freshly churned.

Lemon Curd\sIngredients

• 4 eggs\s• 7 oz. / 200g xylitol\s• ⅓ cup / 2 ½ fl oz. lemon juice (approx. 2 lemons) (approx. 2 lemons) Zest of 1 lemon

• 4 oz. / 110g coconut oil, melted

• 4 oz. / 110g butter, melted Directions

• Whisk the eggs well with a fork and pour into a small pan.

• Add the xylitol, lemon juice, lemon zest, coconut oil, and butter. Whisk ingredients together well.

• Place on the stove over a medium heat and STIR CONSTANTLY as the mixture slowly thickens. It takes 12 – 15 minutes to thicken fully. Embrace it. Be patient.

• DO NOT ALLOW THE MIXTURE TO BOIL – it will curdle, or you will get scrambled eggs.

•

When the mixture is thick enough to coat the back of a spoon, quickly remove it from the heat and pour it through a fine mesh sieve into a glass, lidded container (such as a Pyrex storage bowl) (such as a Pyrex storage bowl). No, you cannot omit this step. It must be sieved!

• Stir the mixture in the sieve until you are left with only the zest pulp and a few strands of egg. Use a second, clean spatula to scrape the underside of the sieve as you go.

• Once all the curd has been passed through the sieve, leave uncovered until completely cold, stirring every 10 minutes to prevent a skin from forming.

• When cold, put the lid on the container and place in the 'fridge. Once chilled it\ will be thick and spreadable.

Peanut Butter Drops\sIngredients

- 1 cup / 8 fl oz. smooth peanut butter, unsweetened 1 TBSP glycerin\s• 1 oz. coconut flour\s• 4 tsp. konjac flour / glucomannan powder Directions

- Leave the jar of peanut butter at room temperature overnight so that it softens.

- Put the peanut butter in a bowl with the glycerin and mix well.

- Sieve the coconut flour and konjac flour together into a separate bowl and mix well.

- Add the mixed flours into the peanut butter in 4 batches, mixing well after each addition.

- When all the flours are well incorporated, cover and place in the 'fridge until the peanut butter stiffens.

-

Line a flat plate with plastic wrap, and pull small pieces of peanut butter out of the bowl and place on the plate. Once all the peanut butter has been divided into little pieces, place the peanut butter drops in the freezer on the plate.

-

Once frozen, if you are storing the peanut butter balls for any length of time before adding them to your ice cream, remove from the plate and place in a glass, airtight container, using greaseproof paper between the layers.

Sneaky peanut butter tip: if you buy peanut butter freshly made from a store that has a peanut butter grinder, you may need to add more coconut and konjac flours to this recipe as this kind of peanut butter tends to be softer than peanut butter in a jar. I used Trader Joe's Smooth Peanut Butter in this recipe. Make sure to check the label if you buy pre-packaged peanut butter. The only ingredients should be peanuts and salt.

Low-Carb Cabbage Casserole\sIngredients

• 2 lbs green cabbage\s• 1 yellow onion\s• 2 garlic cloves

• 4 oz. butter\s• 1½ cups heavy whipping cream\s• 6 tbsp sour cream or crème fraîche

• 6 oz. cream cheese\s• 1 tbsp ranch seasoning

• ½ tsp ground black pepper\s• 1 tsp salt\s• 6 oz. shredded cheese Instructions\s• Preheat the oven to 400°F (200°C). Shred onion, garlic and green cabbage using a sharp knife or a mandolin slicer. The quickest way is to use a food processor.

• Heat a large frying pan and add the butter. Sauté the vegetables until softened, about 8-10 minutes. Add cream, sour cream, cream cheese and spices. Stir thoroughly and let simmer for another 5–10 minutes.

• Add to a greased baking dish. Sprinkle cheese on top and bake for 20 minutes or until the cheese is melted and has turned a golden color.

Tip: These rich flavors pair beautifully with grilled - or fried - meat and fish. Whip up a double batch, and freeze the extra in small containers for a quick side dish any night of the week. Save even more time by using pre-shredded coleslaw – just avoid mixes with carrots if you can.

Low-Carb Zucchini And Walnut Salad\sIngredients Dressing

• 2 tbsp olive oil\s• ¾ cup mayonnaise or vegan mayonnaise

• 2 tsp lemon juice

• 1 garlic clove, finely minced\s• ½ tsp salt

- ¼ tsp chili powder Salad\s• 1 head of Romaine lettuce\s• 4 oz. arugula lettuce

- ¼ cup finely chopped fresh chives or scallions

- 2 zucchini\s• 1 tbsp olive oil

- salt and pepper

- 3½ oz. chopped walnuts or pecans Instructions

- In a small bowl, whisk together all ingredients for the dressing. Reserve the dressing to develop flavor while you make the salad.

-

Trim and cut the salad. Place the Romaine, arugula and chives in a large bowl.

- Split the zucchini length-wise and scoop out the seeds. Cut the zucchini halves crosswise into half-inch pieces.

- Heat olive oil in a frying pan over medium heat, until it shimmers. Add zucchini to the pan, and season with salt and pepper. Sauté until lightly browned but still firm.

• Add the cooked zucchini to the salad, and mix together.

• Roast the nuts briefly in the same pan as the zucchini. Season with salt and pepper. Spoon nuts onto salad, and drizzle with salad dressing.

Tip: Let your imagination soar! This dressing pairs beautifully with other salads – or even as a refreshingly cool sauce for meat or fish. Make up extra dressing to keep on hand. The zucchini salad is super flexible too! Try it as the perfect base for hearty grilled beef, chicken or fish. It stores well for at least 5 days in the refrigerator.

Low-Carb Broccoli Mash\sIngredients

• 1½ lbs broccoli\s• 4 tbsp fresh basil or fresh parsley, finely chopped\s• 3 oz. butter

• 1 garlic clove\s• salt and pepper Instructions\s• Chop the broccoli into florets and peel and cut the stem into small pieces. Boil the broccoli in plenty of lightly salted water for a couple of minutes – just enough to retain a somewhat firm texture. Discard the water.\s• Blend with the other ingredients in a food processor or use an immersion blender.

- Salt and pepper to taste.

- Add more oil or butter if you so desire.

- Serve piping hot!

Tip: You can use either frozen or fresh broccoli with this recipe. If you use fresh broccoli, save the stalk, peel it with a sharp knife and slice thinly. Cut the rest of the broccoli into smaller florets of roughly equal size. Feel free to substitute olive oil for some of the butter in any proportion you choose.

Cauliflower Mac and Cheese\sServes 6, Prep time: 10 minutes, Cook time: 4 to 6 hours on low, 2 to 3 hours on high

Macaroni and cheese lovers rejoice! When you swap out the pasta and use cauliflower, you're left with a low-carb taste sensation that is creamy and filling. It makes great leftovers and the kids will like it, too. If the sauce seems too thick after it's finished cooking, stir in a little water or vegetable broth.

Ingredients\s• 2 medium heads cauliflower, cut into small florets

- 1 small onion, diced

- 3 cups Cheese Sauce Direction

- Coat a slow cooker generously with cooking spray.

-

Add the cauliflower and onion to the slow cooker.

- Pour the cheese sauce over the top.\s• Cook on low for 4 to 6 hours or on high for 2 to 3 hours, or until the cauliflower is tender.

Balsamic And Bacon Vegetable Medley\sServes 4, Prep time: 15 minutes, Cook time: 4 to 6 hours on low, 2 to 3 hours on high.

Here is a side dish perfect for summer, when these vegetables will be at their freshest and most flavorful. By cooking in a slow cooker, you don't need to stand over a hot stove. Feel free to swap in whatever veggies you like the best. And it's never wrong to add a little extra bacon.

Ingredients\s• 8 ounces bacon, cooked and crumbled

• 1 small onion, chopped\s• 2 bell peppers, seeded and chopped\s• 3 ounces carrots, peeled and chopped

• 3 ounces green beans, cut into 1-inch pieces

• 3 ounces Brussels sprouts, trimmed and halved

• 3 ounces beets, peeled and chopped\s• 3 ounces summer squash or zucchini, chopped\s• ¼ cup water

• 1 tablespoon extra-virgin olive oil\s• 2 tablespoons balsamic vinegar Direction

• Coat a slow cooker generously with cooking spray.

•

Add the bacon, onion, bell peppers, carrots, green beans, Brussels sprouts, beets, and squash to the slow cooker.

• In a small bowl, mix together the water, olive oil, and vinegar to make a sauce. Pour it over the top of the vegetables.

•

Cook on low for 4 to 6 hours or on high for 2 to 3 hours, or until Brussels sprouts are tender.

Garden Vegetable Soup\sServes 4, Prep time: 10 minutes, Cook time: 6 to 8 hours on low, 3 to 4 hours on high.

Grab your favorite vegetables for this super easy soup that is friendly for almost any healthy eating lifestyle: paleo, Whole30, vegetarian, vegan—it's a real diet pleaser. I love the combination of vegetables I've included below, but don't let that fence you in. Swap in whatever you find in the store that's fresh and low-carb. Try yellow squash instead of zucchini, or asparagus instead of green beans. Choose sturdy vegetables that won't turn to mush during the long cook time.

Ingredients\s• 4 cups Vegetable Broth or store-bought low-sodium vegetable broth

• 1 (15-ounce) can low-sodium or no-salt-added diced tomatoes

• 2 small zucchini, diced\s• 2 carrots, peeled and chopped

• 4 ounces green beans, chopped

- 4 ounces kale, chopped

- 1 onion, diced

- 1 bell pepper, seeded and diced\s• 2 garlic cloves, minced

- 1 tablespoon Italian seasoning\s• ½ teaspoon salt

- ¼ teaspoon freshly ground black pepper\s• 1 bay leaf Direction

- Add the broth, tomatoes, zucchini, carrots, green beans, kale, onion, bell pepper, garlic, Italian seasoning, salt, black pepper, and bay leaf to a slow cooker.

- Cook on low for 6 to 8 hours or on high for 3 to 4 hours, or until vegetables are soft.

- Remove the bay leaf prior to serving.

Blueberry Muffin Cake\sServes 10, Prep time: 15 minutes, Cook time: 4 to 6 hours on low, 2 to 3 hours on high.

Is this a cake or a muffin? It's both. Serve this sweet, keto-friendly blueberry treat as an after- dinner dessert or as part of your next brunch spread.

Ingredient\s• 3 cups almond flour

• ½ cup 2 percent fat plain Greek yogurt

• ¼ cup powdered erythritol sweetener of your choice\s• 3 large eggs

• 2 to 3 teaspoons grated lemon zest\s• 1½ teaspoons baking powder

• 1 teaspoon vanilla extract\s• ½ teaspoon baking soda\s• ¼ teaspoon salt

• 1 cup fresh or frozen blueberries Direction

• Coat a slow cooker generously with cooking spray.

•

In a large bowl, mix together the almond flour, yogurt, erythritol, eggs, lemon zest, baking powder, vanilla, baking soda, and salt until well blended. Carefully fold in the blueberries.

• Pour the batter into the slow cooker.

• Place a paper towel between the slow cooker and the lid to cut down on any condensation that develops. Cook on low for 4 to 6 hours or on high for 2 to 3 hours, or until a toothpick inserted in the center comes out clean.

Pecan Cookie\sServes 8, Prep time: 10 minutes, Cook time: 4 to 6 hours on low, 2 to 3 hours on high

This will remind you of a buttery pecan sandie, but you can enjoy it guilt-free. It's another great option if you're following a keto diet, too.

Ingredient\s• 1¼ cup almond flour

• ⅔ cup powdered erythritol sweetener of your choice\s• ⅓ cup chopped pecans\s• 1 large egg

• 5 tbsp unsalted butter, room temp

• 1 tablespoon shredded coconut

• 1 teaspoon powdered sugar

Directions: 12 teaspoon vanilla extract

• Spray a slow cooker with cooking spray liberally.

•

Mix the almond flour, erythritol, pecans, egg, butter, coconut flour, baking powder, and vanilla in a large mixing bowl until well combined. In a slow cooker, pour the batter in.

•

To reduce the amount of condensation that forms, place a paper towel between the slow cooker and the lid. Cook 4 to 6 hours on low or 2 to 3 hours on high, or until a toothpick inserted in the middle comes out clean.

Serves 8 / Asparagus and Cauliflower Hash Cooking time: 6 to 8 hours on low, 3 to 4 hours on high, prep time: 10 minutes

Asparagus is high in vitamins A and C and is a rich source of fiber. If you're monitoring your blood sugar, it's an excellent veggie to select. Cauliflower has risen in popularity as a low-carb alternative to rice and potatoes. You won't be able to tell it's not potatoes if you use it to create hash browns with the cheese and eggs. Spray for cooking

• 12 big eggs, peeled and halved

• 1 teaspoon salt • 12 cup low-fat 1% milk • 2 cups shredded part-skim mozzarella cheese

1 medium head cauliflower, shredded or riced • 14 teaspoon freshly ground black pepper

Directions: • 1 pound chopped asparagus

• Spray a slow cooker with cooking spray liberally.

• Beat the eggs, milk, cheese, salt, and pepper together in a large mixing basin.

• In the slow cooker's bottom, place half of the cauliflower. Half of the asparagus should be placed on top of the dish. Carry on with the rest of the cauliflower and asparagus in the same manner.

•

In a slow cooker, crack the eggs.

• Cook for 6 to 8 hours on low or 3 to 4 hours on high, or until the eggs are set.

Quiche with Broccoli, Bacon, and Cheese serves eight people. 5 minute prep time 6–8 hours on low, 3–4 hours on high

Is there such a thing as a crustless quiche? The delightfully buttery and flaky quiche crust is irresistible, but this dish has so much flavor that you won't miss it. Remove the bacon and replace it with your favorite extra veggies if you're a vegetarian. Zucchini, onions, and mushrooms are among the vegetables I like. 8 big eggs, sprayed with cooking spray

• 12 cup grated Parmesan cheese • 2 cups reduced-fat 2% milk

• 2 lbs. thawed frozen broccoli florets

• Cooked and crumbled bacon (6 ounces)

• 34 cup medium shredded Cheddar cheese, split

• Spray a slow cooker with cooking spray liberally.

• Beat the eggs, milk, Parmesan, and salt together in a medium mixing basin.

In the slow cooker, combine the broccoli, bacon, and half the Cheddar cheese. In a separate bowl, whisk together the eggs and milk. The remaining Cheddar cheese should be sprinkled over the top.

•

Cook for 6 to 8 hours on low or 3 to 4 hours on high, or until the eggs are firm.

8 servings granola 10 minute prep time Time to cook: 6 hours on low and 3 hours on high.

Granola normally doesn't come to mind when you think about low-carb foods. Most people also believe that store-bought granola is healthful, so they avoid making their own. Unfortunately, a lot of store-bought granola is coated in—wait for it—sugar. sugar. Fortunately, this low-carb version is simple to prepare (and delicious), and you have complete control over the ingredients, ensuring that they are all natural and free of fillers.

Ingredients

• Almonds, 212 cup

• 14 cup chia seeds • 12 cup dried berries • 14 cup unsweetened coconut flakes

12 teaspoon salt 1 teaspoon cinnamon

1 teaspoon vanilla • 14 teaspoon nutmeg • 14 cup coconut oil Direction

• Using cooking spray, coat the sides of a slow cooker.

• In a slow cooker, mix together the almonds, coconut flakes, dried berries, chia seeds, cinnamon, salt, and nutmeg.

•

Melt the coconut oil in a medium-sized bowl. Add the vanilla extract and whisk to combine.

-

Pour the mixture into the slow cooker and stir to thoroughly moisten all of the ingredients.

- Make a barrier between the slow cooker and the lid by placing a small towel or two paper towels between them. This will keep the granola from becoming wet while it cooks. If the condensation isn't caught, the granola will get soggy.

- Cook for 6 hours on low or 3 hours on high, depending on your preference.

- To chill the granola, spread it out on a baking pan.• 5 tbsp unsalted butter, room temp

- 1 tablespoon shredded coconut

- 1 teaspoon powdered sugar

Directions: 12 teaspoon vanilla extract

- Spray a slow cooker with cooking spray liberally.

-

Mix the almond flour, erythritol, pecans, egg, butter, coconut flour, baking powder, and vanilla in a large mixing bowl until well combined. In a slow cooker, pour the batter in.

•

To reduce the amount of condensation that forms, place a paper towel between the slow cooker and the lid. Cook 4 to 6 hours on low or 2 to 3 hours on high, or until a toothpick inserted in the middle comes out clean.

Serves 8 / Asparagus and Cauliflower Hash Cooking time: 6 to 8 hours on low, 3 to 4 hours on high, prep time: 10 minutes

Asparagus is high in vitamins A and C and is a rich source of fiber. If you're monitoring your blood sugar, it's an excellent veggie to select. Cauliflower has risen in popularity as a low-carb alternative to rice and potatoes. You won't be able to tell it's not potatoes if you use it to create hash browns with the cheese and eggs. Spray for cooking

• 12 big eggs, peeled and halved

• 1 teaspoon salt • 12 cup low-fat 1% milk • 2 cups shredded part-skim mozzarella cheese

1 medium head cauliflower, shredded or riced • 14 teaspoon freshly ground black pepper

Directions: • 1 pound chopped asparagus

• Spray a slow cooker with cooking spray liberally.

• Beat the eggs, milk, cheese, salt, and pepper together in a large mixing basin.

• In the slow cooker's bottom, place half of the cauliflower. Half of the asparagus should be placed on top of the dish. Carry on with the rest of the cauliflower and asparagus in the same manner.

•

In a slow cooker, crack the eggs.

• Cook for 6 to 8 hours on low or 3 to 4 hours on high, or until the eggs are set.

Quiche with Broccoli, Bacon, and Cheese serves eight people. 5 minute prep time 6–8 hours on low, 3–4 hours on high

Is there such a thing as a crustless quiche? The delightfully buttery and flaky quiche crust is irresistible, but this dish has so much flavor that you won't miss it. Remove the bacon and replace it with your favorite extra veggies if you're a vegetarian. Zucchini, onions, and mushrooms are among the vegetables I like. 8 big eggs, sprayed with cooking spray

• 12 cup grated Parmesan cheese • 2 cups reduced-fat 2% milk

• 2 lbs. thawed frozen broccoli florets

• Cooked and crumbled bacon (6 ounces)

• 34 cup medium shredded Cheddar cheese, split

• Spray a slow cooker with cooking spray liberally.

• Beat the eggs, milk, Parmesan, and salt together in a medium mixing basin.

In the slow cooker, combine the broccoli, bacon, and half the Cheddar cheese. In a separate bowl, whisk together the eggs and milk. The remaining Cheddar cheese should be sprinkled over the top.

•

Cook for 6 to 8 hours on low or 3 to 4 hours on high, or until the eggs are firm.

8 servings granola 10 minute prep time Time to cook: 6 hours on low and 3 hours on high.

Granola normally doesn't come to mind when you think about low-carb foods. Most people also believe that store-bought granola is healthful, so they avoid making their own. Unfortunately, a lot of store-bought granola is coated in—wait for it—sugar. sugar. Fortunately, this low-carb version is simple to prepare (and delicious), and you have complete control over the ingredients, ensuring that they are all natural and free of fillers.

Ingredients

• Almonds, 212 cup

• 14 cup chia seeds • 12 cup dried berries • 14 cup unsweetened coconut flakes

12 teaspoon salt 1 teaspoon cinnamon

1 teaspoon vanilla • 14 teaspoon nutmeg • 14 cup coconut oil Direction

• Using cooking spray, coat the sides of a slow cooker.

• In a slow cooker, mix together the almonds, coconut flakes, dried berries, chia seeds, cinnamon, salt, and nutmeg.

•

Melt the coconut oil in a medium-sized bowl. Add the vanilla extract and whisk to combine.

•

Pour the mixture into the slow cooker and stir to thoroughly moisten all of the ingredients.

• Make a barrier between the slow cooker and the lid by placing a small towel or two paper towels between them. This will keep the granola from becoming wet while it cooks. If the condensation isn't caught, the granola will get soggy.

• Cook for 6 hours on low or 3 hours on high, depending on your preference.

• To chill the granola, spread it out on a baking pan.

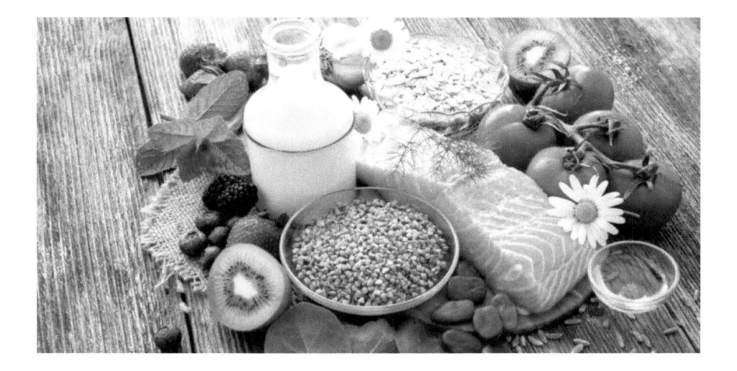

CPSIA information can be obtained
at www.ICGtesting.com
Printed in the USA
LVHW020851290122
709722LV00007B/268